sofien Kamoun
imtinene Ben Mrad

Early complications of pacemakers and defibrillators

sofien Kamoun
imtinene Ben Mrad

Early complications of pacemakers and defibrillators

ScienciaScripts

Imprint

Any brand names and product names mentioned in this book are subject to trademark, brand or patent protection and are trademarks or registered trademarks of their respective holders. The use of brand names, product names, common names, trade names, product descriptions etc. even without a particular marking in this work is in no way to be construed to mean that such names may be regarded as unrestricted in respect of trademark and brand protection legislation and could thus be used by anyone.

Cover image: www.ingimage.com

This book is a translation from the original published under ISBN 978-613-8-43195-4.

Publisher:
Sciencia Scripts
is a trademark of
Dodo Books Indian Ocean Ltd., member of the OmniScriptum S.R.L Publishing group
str. A.Russo 15, of. 61, Chisinau-2068, Republic of Moldova Europe
Printed at: see last page
ISBN: 978-620-4-06991-3

TITLE: EARLY COMPLICATIONS OF PACEMAKERS AND DEFIBRILLATORS

1

TABLE OF CONTENTS

LIST OF FIGURES

LIST OF ABBREVIATIONS

AAP: Anti-platelet agent

AVK : Anti-vitamin K

AVB: atrioventricular block

COPD: chronic obstructive pulmonary disease

CEP: cephalic

CRT: cardiac resynchronization therapy

ICD: automatic implantable defibrillator

SD: sinus dysfunction

DM: Diabetes mellitus

ECG: electrocardiogram

LVEF: left ventricular ejection fraction

UFH: unfractionated heparin

HTA: high blood pressure

CKD: chronic renal failure

NYHA: New York Heart Association

OR: Odds Ratio

PM: pacemaker

PNO: Pneumothorax

SC: subclavian

TE: thrombo-embolic

INTRODUCTION

Permanent cardiac pacing is one of the most important medical innovations of the 20th century. Although initially designed for the prevention of sudden death from syncopal complete atrioventricular block (AVB) (Stokes-Adams attacks), sinus dysfunction is now the most posited indication for permanent pacemaker implantation worldwide [1]. In the USA, sinus dysfunction has become the main indication for pacemaker implantation in over 50% of patients [1]. Indications have expanded beyond symptomatic bradycardia and now include neuro-cardiogenic syncope, obstructive hypertrophic cardiomyopathy, and cardiac resynchronization therapy (CRT) for congestive heart failure. The role of atrial pacing in the prevention of atrial fibrillation (AF) is not yet validated [2-6].Thanks to continuous technical progress, the modalities and objectives of cardiac pacing have changed radically since the first implantation in 1958 by Senning & Elmquist [7]. At that time, pacing was performed by the epicardial route (in an asynchronous mode). It was not until the 1970s that endocavitary sentinel pacing was introduced. In the 1980s, cardiac pacing and defibrillation underwent a real technological upheaval with the advent of dual-chamber pacemakers, restoring efficient atrial function and thus obtaining physiological atrioventricular synchrony. Currently, the objectives of cardiac stimulation are much more physiological and ambitious, aiming at quality of life and a better adaptation to exercise. In the 90s, biventricular resynchronization was born, coupled or not with cardiac defibrillation function.it is however obvious that these goals can only be reached on the condition of an individual optimization of the pacing mode, through a very precise pre and postoperative evaluation of the particular needs of each patient.on the other hand, this therapy remains burdened by a complication rate which, despite the therapeutic and technological advances, has remained stable for several years. The follow-up of implanted patients also suffers from several shortcomings concerning on the one hand the modalities of this follow-up and on the other hand the management of the complications inherent to this therapy.This technique has been the subject of several publications dictating the rules of prescription of cardiac stimulation and analyzing, with the hindsight available at present, its benefits and its risks [1,2].In Tunisia, cardiac stimulation has been in existence for more than 40 years, and cardiac defibrillation for almost 25 years. Several Tunisian authors such as Mourali in 1997 [8], Hajlaoui in 2000 [9], Ben Ameur in 2001 [10], Slimane in 2002 [11] and Sdiri in 2013 [12] have conducted studies on cardiac pacing by identifying the main complications. However, in the absence of a national cardiac pacing registry, it is delicate to count the number of implantations per year, and the number of early and late complications inherent to the procedure of fitting with cardiac pacing and defibrillation devices.In this perspective, we are interested in estimating the prevalence of complications of cardiac stimulation and defibrillation during the first 30 days following the implantation procedure and this through the experience of our cardiology department of the Habib Thameur hospital, to undertake a comparison between the complications related to pacemakers and automatic implantable defibrillators and to possibly search for the factors associated with these complications

METHODS

I- Type of study and study population:

This was a retrospective, descriptive, repeated cross-sectional and analytical study of 441 patients collected in the cardiology department of HABIB THAMEUR hospital, between January 2011 and January 2018, who were consecutively implanted with a pacemaker (PM) or an automatic implantable defibrillator (ICD) all indications combined.

II- Study objectives:

The objectives of our study were:

- To estimate the prevalence of complications in the first 30 days following a pacemaker or implantable cardioverter defibrillator device,
- Compare the complication rate according to the device implanted,

- Look for factors that predict these complications.

III- Population :

1- Inclusion criteria:

We included all patients fitted during the period between January 2011 and January 2018 with a :

- Pacemaker in primary implantation including single, double and triple chamber,
- Cardiac defibrillator in primary implantation including single, double and triple chambers,
- Change of pacemaker or automatic implantable defibrillator device

whether or not it is associated with a probe change.

2- Exclusion and non-inclusion criteria :

o Change of pacemaker lead or implantable automatic defibrillator without changing the box. These were two patients who were not implanted in the department and who had a lead-related complication requiring this change.

IV- Collection of clinical and procedural data:

From the data available in the medical records and in the operative reports, and during the length of stay after implantation, we collected the following:

1- Epidemiological and clinical data:

- Age and gender

- Cardiovascular history and risk factors:

❖ Type 1 or type 2 diabetes, how long it has been present and the treatment prescribed. Diabetes was defined by two fasting blood glucose levels above 1.26 g/l and/or a glycosylated hemoglobin above 6.2%.

❖ High blood pressure (HBP), how long it has been present and the treatment prescribed, with high blood pressure defined as systolic blood pressure greater than or equal to 140mmHg and/or diastolic blood pressure greater than or equal to 90mmHg.

❖ Dyslipidemia: defined as elevated cholesterol and/or triglyceride levels (greater than 2g/l and greater than 1.5 g/l respectively)

❖ Active smoking. Past smoking has not been studied.

❖ Chronic renal failure defined by creatinine clearance

less than 60 ml/min according to MDRD formula.

❖ History of coronary artery disease or myocardial revascularization procedure.
- History of ischemic stroke (transient or acute)

constituted),

- History of heart failure,

- History of valve disease or surgery

- History of ventricular or supra-ventricular rhythm (fibrillation and atrial flutter),
- The drug treatments administered to patients, including the use of

anticoagulants and antiplatelet agents during the perioperative phase,

- Symptoms on admission: syncope, lipothymia, chest pain, dyspnea (classified according to NYHA) and palpitations.

- Signs of heart failure on admission
- Electrocardiogram data during hospitalization,
- Ultrasound LVEF according to Simpson's method

- For pacemakers: The type of conductive disorder (sino-atrial or atrioventricular) and the selected diagnosis.
- For automatic implantable defibrillators: indication in primary or secondary prevention.

2- Data related to the implementation procedure :

a. Stimulators and probes :

- Type of probe (active or passive), bipolar or multipolar, monocoil or double coil for defibrillation probes,
- Site of fixation (DO: right atrium, RV: right ventricle, LV: left ventricle)

- Number of probes

- Pace maker case with one, two or three probe connector,

- Defibrillator housing with single, dual or triple lead connector and IS1-DF1 or DF-4 connector.

b. Implementation process :

o **For primary implantation :**

► Implantation is done in the cardiac catheterization room before the

coronary angiography,

► The room is disinfected the day before the procedure by the Phagogene,

► The paramedical team consists of two nurses or one nurse and one anesthesia technician,
► Shaving of the surgical site if there is an indication, 24 hours before the procedure,

► Checking the haemostasis and platelet count the day before the procedure. An INR of less than 3 is imperative for the procedure. If an INR>3 is imperative (mitral prosthesis), heparin therapy with an electric syringe is instituted, with monitoring of the aPTT twice a day, and the heparin therapy is stopped two hours before the procedure and restarted 4 hours after the procedure is completed,

► The patient is premedicated with Atarax before the procedure, 50 mg the day before the implantation and 50 mg two hours before the implantation,

► The patient is placed on the operating table and given 1g of pro-paracetamol by slow infusion, combined with morphine sulphate by subcutaneous or intravenous titration and metoclopramide, depending on the patient's condition,

► For patients who are bradycardic, an infusion of Isuprel with an electric syringe pump is done to allow a heart rate of about 40bpm,

► First disinfection of the surgical site with Betadine, disinfecting the homo-lateral axillary hollow,

► The implant physician performs a surgical wash with Betadine foam for 10 minutes,

► For the implantation of pacemakers or triple-chamber defibrillators, a second physician assists the implanting physician in the procedure,

► Preparation of the instrument table for the operator,

► Placement of a tissue or single-use surgical drape, covering the entire patient and the operating table and separating the patient's face from the surgical site. This drape is perforated exposing the surgical site,

► Second disinfection with Betadine,

► Local anesthesia with 2% Xylocaine,

► Surgical incision in the delto-pectoral fold,

► At the time of incision, the patient received 1g of Cefapirine (Cefaloject) in case of no allergy to cephalosporins or multi-allergic terrain. Only one patient allergic to cephalosporins received 400 mg of Teicoplanin,

► Dissection of the subcutaneous and muscular planes with a Guyot forceps without

the use of an electric scalpel or scissors,

► Systematic cephalic approach, except for patients in complete sino-atrial or atrioventricular block on Isuprel,

► Stripping the cephalic vein, puncturing it and inserting the first probe, or alternatively, advancing a 0.036 J guidewire over which a peelable desilet is advanced,

► If the cephalic vein approach fails, or if it is not indicated, a keyboard approach is performed: puncture of the subclavian vein and placement of a 0.036 guidewire on which a peelable stent is placed, the distal end of which is positioned at the level of the superior vena cava. This puncture is performed for the first attempt without radiological control, and if unsuccessful, the puncture is performed under fluoroscopy,

► The ventricular lead is first advanced and is fixed with predilection at the apex, more rarely on the interventricular septum,

► This entire procedure is repeated in the same way for the atrial lead, with optimal positioning at the level of the right atrium, or failing that on the lateral wall of the right atrium. Only one patient with sinus dysfunction and extensive atrial fibrosis required the fixation of the lead on the
interatrial septum. The progression of the atrial probe can be done by cephalic way, or under ipsilateral clavière,

► For the left ventricular lead, the approach is systematically under the left keyboard. A specialized curved sheath is advanced to catheterize the ostium of the coronary sinus, through which a guide will be advanced to catheterize a coronary venous branch, lateral or posterolateral, in which the dedicated lead for left ventricular stimulation will be positioned,

► Preparation of the box of the device implanted in intrapectoral or retropectoral,

► Careful hemostasis during the preparation of the dressing room,

► Checking impedances and stimulation thresholds and probe detection,

► Ligation of the cephalic vein if it has been approached,

► Fixation of the probes to the muscular or aponeurotic plane by a non-absorbable thread,

► Connection of the probes to the box which will be placed in its box,

► Checking for hemostasis,

► The fascia, subcutaneous and cutaneous planes are closed with absorbable sutures for both planes and with non-absorbable sutures for the skin. The suture of the cutaneous plane is of the intradermal type for young patients, using an absorbable thread,

► The procedure is completed by taking an x-ray of the entire chest to

check the position of the probe(s) and the absence of pneumothorax

► Compression bandage to be kept on for 48 hours.

o **For relocation :**

► Same procedure for preparing the patient for the installation,

► The incision is made directly above the explanted case,

► Dissection with Guyot forceps, extraction of the case and disconnection of the probes

► Checking the probes. If their stimulation and detection parameters

are accepted, the probes are kept if not they are substituted.

► Apart from the infection, the catheters are not extracted, but abandoned. A silicone cap is placed on the proximal end of the abandoned catheter to prevent mechanical erosion,

► The new box is connected to the probe(s), which will be placed in the same box

of the former botier,

► No instillation of Rifamycin into the lodge,

► Closure of the aponeurotic, subcutaneous and cutaneous planes with absorbable suture for both planes and with non-absorbable suture for the skin. No intradermal suture in this case.

c. **Immediate postoperative data**

• The duration of the procedure,

• Prescription of an antibiotic prophylaxis (systematic for all patients based on Cefapirin 1g every 8 hours or failing that 400mg of Teicoplanin per day for a minimum of 48h).

• The thermal curve,

• Electrocardiographic monitoring and search for a rhythm disorder,

• The search for a stimulation and detection defect,

• Examination of the surgical site for signs of infection (wound

inflammatory, pus discharge, loose sutures),

• Chest X-ray data in bed on the day of implantation and again in

standing position 48 hours later,

- The search for thromboembolic complications : thromboembolic disease or pulmonary embolism.
- The search for hematoma,
- Death: cause and delay in relation to implantation,
- Anti-vitamin K is taken again in the evening of the same day of the implantation.

3- Clinical events during the first 30 days following implantation

o The nature of the complication: We considered the following events as complications:

o Pneumothorax, defined by a gaseous pleural effusion. It is considered as total if the detachment has occurred on the whole visceral layer of the pleura and partial if it has involved a portion of this serosa,

o Infection defined by inflammatory signs of the lodge associated with a

often purulent discharge from the scar with fever,

o Endocarditis on catheter is defined as:

■ The combination of 3 of the following criteria: fever, positive blood cultures, visualization of vegetations or thickening of the tube on transesophageal ultrasound, septic pulmonary embolism,

■ Or culture of the extracted probe positive

o The hematoma defined by a bloody effusion at the level of the lodge putting in tension the sutures of the scar,

o Venous thromboembolic disease: defined as deep vein thrombosis of any topography and/or pulmonary embolism,

o Cardiac perforation: defined by a break in continuity of one of the

the cardiac walls secondary to a trauma of the latter by a probe,

o Lead displacement: defined by a defect in pacing and/or detection of ventricular or atrial activity confirmed by chest X-ray showing a change in the position of the lead compared to its initial implantation site, with or without functional signs (syncope, lipothymia, dyspnea)

o Death of any cause,

o We have not had any cases of phrenic or pectoral stimulation.

o Complication day,

o Length of hospitalization.

V- Statistical analysis:

Data were entered and analyzed using SPSS® version 22.0

1- Descriptive study :

Simple frequencies and relative frequencies (percentages) were calculated for categorical variables. Means, standard deviations, and extreme values were calculated for quantitative variables with a normal distribution, and medians, interquartile range, and extreme values were calculated for quantitative variables whose distribution deviated from normality. The normality test used was the Shapiro-Wilk test. The distribution was considered normal if this test was insignificant, and the hypothesis of normality was rejected if it was not.

2- Analytical study :

We subdivided our patient population into two groups: Group A: without complicationGroup B: with complication.

A- Comparison of averages :

The comparison of 2 means on independent series was performed using the two-tailed Student's t-test for independent series for quantitative variables with normal distribution and the two-tailed Mann-Witney U test in the opposite case. The significance level was set at $p<0.05$.

B- Comparison of percentages :

The comparison of percentages on independent series was performed by the two-tailed Pearson's Chi-2 test, and by the two-tailed Fisher's exact test according to the validity conditions. The significance level was set at $p<0.05$.

C- Search for event predictive factors :

a} Univariate study:

The search for factors predictive of complication was performed by comparing the means or medians of each group for quantitative variables and the percentages for qualitative variables according to the modalities in paragraphs V-2-A and B.

b} Multivariate study:

To identify independent predictors of complications, we used a stepwise logistic regression model with maximum likelihood. We introduced all factors with a significance level "p" less than 0.05 in univariate and bivariate analysis, and then added gender, age and factors with a significance level greater than 0.05 but less than 0.20. The independent factors retained were those with an adjusted significance level of less than 0.05 and when no p was less than 0.05, the most significant factor with a p between 0.05 and 0.10 was retained.

I - DESCRIPTIVE STUDY :

We conducted a retrospective, descriptive, repeated cross-sectional and analytical study of 441 patients collected in the cardiology department of HABIB THAMEUR hospital, between January 2011 and January 2018, who were consecutively implanted with a pacemaker (PM) or an automatic implantable defibrillator (ICD) all indications combined.

The locations were distributed as follows:

- first-time implantation :
- 102 single-chamber pacemakers, all ventricular
- 233 dual-chamber pacemakers. No dual-chamber pacemakers.
- 2 triple-chamber pacemakers, both with a complete block of the left branch (QRS>160ms),
- 23 single-chamber defibrillators,
- 46 dual-chamber defibrillators,
- 10 triple-chamber defibrillators, all with a complete block of the left branch (QRS>140ms),

- Change of case :
- Seven single-chamber pacemakers, all ventricular,
- 15 dual-chamber pacemakers. No dual-chamber pacemakers,
- No triple-chamber pacemaker,
- A single-chamber defibrillator,
- A double-chamber defibrillator,
- A triple chamber defibrillator.

The indications for defibrillator fitting were:
- 50 in primary prevention, divided into :

o 41 patients with ischemic cardiomyopathy,

o seven patients with non-ischemic dilated cardiomyopathy, including two with valves,

o two patients with hypertrophic cardiomyopathy,

- 32 in secondary prevention, divided into :

o 12 patients with non-ischemic dilated cardiomyopathy,

o 12 patients with ischemic heart disease

o Four patients with arrhythmogenic right ventricular dysplasia

o Two patients with hypertrophic cardiomyopathy

o Brugada syndrome

o idiopathic ventricular fibrillation

1- Epidemiological characteristics :

1.1- Age :

The mean age of the study population was 66.5 ± 11.1 years with extremes ranging from 31 to 97 years. Patients over 70 years of age represented 36.3% (Figure 1).

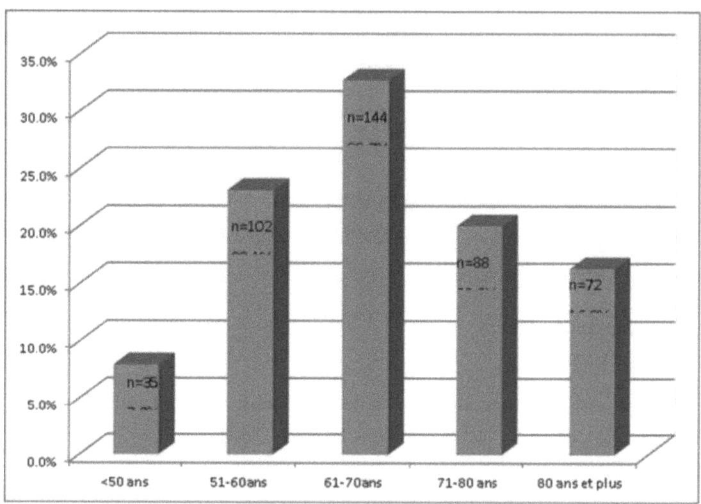

Figure 1: Distribution of patients by age group

1.2- Gender :

Our population consisted of 236 men (53.5%) and 205 women (46.5%).

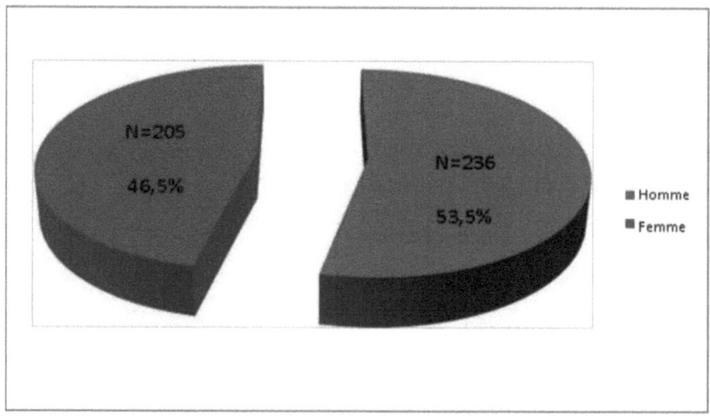

Figure 2: Gender distribution

1.3- Background :

a- Diabetes:

Diabetes was found in 238 patients (54.0%) in the study population. Type 2 diabetes was present in all cases. In this population of diabetics, 56% were on oral anti-diabetics and 44% were insulin-requiring.

b- High blood pressure:

Hypertension was found in 286 patients (64.9%) of the patient population studied.

c- Smoking:

149 patients (33.8%) were active smokers with a clear male predominance (79.2% vs 20.8%).

d- Dyslipidemia:

Dyslipidemia was found in 130 patients, i.e. in 29.5% of cases. It was distributed in a similar way according to gender (50% vs 50%).

e- Chronic renal failure

Chronic renal failure was found in 13 patients (2.9%), only two of whom were on hemodialysis. It was distributed in a similar way according to gender (53.8% in men and 46.2% in women).

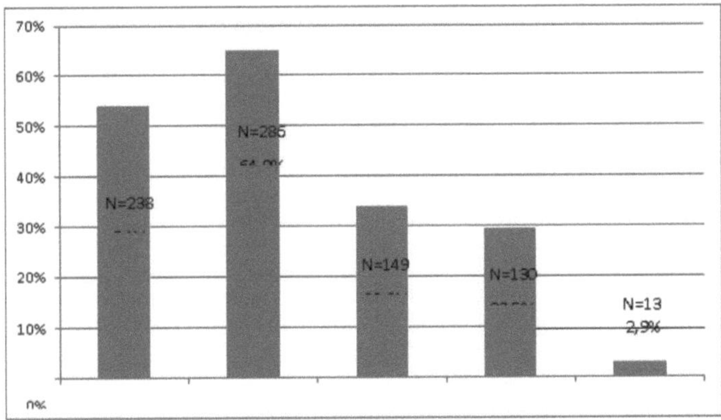

Figure 3: Frequency of the different cardiovascular risk factors in our population

f- Vascular, rhythmic, valvular and bronchopulmonary history:

• A history of coronary artery disease was found in 110 patients (25.0%) with a similar gender distribution (59 men to 51 women) in our population,

- A history of ischemic stroke or transient ischemic attack was found in 21 patients (2.9%),

- Valve disease was found in 38 patients (8.6%). 21 patients (4.8%) had a mechanical valve prosthesis, similarly divided between aortic (10 patients) and mitral (11 patients).
- Emboligenic supraventricular rhythm disorders (atrial fibrillation (AF) and flutter) were reported in 62 patients (14.1%). AF was observed in 56 patients (12.7%). Ventricular rhythm disorders were found in only 6 patients or 1.4% of our study population.
- A history of COPD was noted in 17 patients, i.e. 3.9% of our population.

1.5- Clinical data :

a- Functional symptomatology :

- In our work, 225 patients (51.7% of cases) presented with symptoms on admission. These were mainly lipothymia in 50.6% of cases and syncope in 24.5% of cases.

- Table 2 summarizes the signs and percentages of these signs on admission

Table I: Symptoms on admission

SYMPTOMS	Number of patients (%}
Lipothymia	223 (50,6%)
Syncope	108 (24,5%)
Stress dyspnea (NYHA II and III)	173 (39,2%)
Palpitations	9 (2,0%)
Resting dyspnea (NYHA IV)	22 (5,0%)
Chest pain	13 (2,9%)
No symptoms	66 (15,0%)

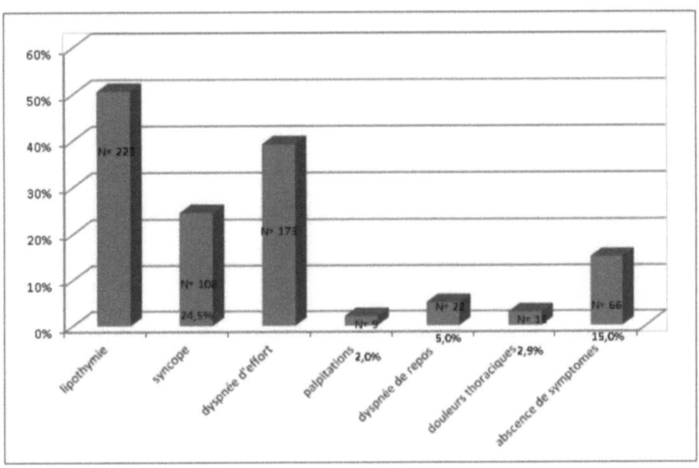

Figure 4: Distribution of symptoms at admission

b- Physical signs:

The physical examination on admission was unremarkable in 145 patients (32.9%). 51 patients (11.6%) had signs of congestive heart failure. 32 patients (7.3%) had a murmur (systolic and/or diastolic) on auscultation 213 patients (48.3%) had other features on clinical examination unrelated to their cardiac pathology

1.6- Electrocardiographic data at admission :

- 379 patients (85.9%) were in sinus rhythm on admission,

- Atrial fibrillation was noted in 56 patients or 12.7%,

- 6 patients (1.4%) had atrial flutter,

- 24 patients had bradyarrhythmia (5.4%),

- 36 patients had second degree atrioventricular block (8.2%),

- Third degree atrioventricular block in 215 patients (48.6%),

- Sinus dysfunction (sino-atrial block and/or atrial rhythmic disease and

and/or chronotropic insufficiency) in 82 patients (18.6%),

- Complete left bundle branch block with QRS >160ms in 13 patients (2.9%).

1.7- Left ventricular ejection fraction :

The median LVEF was 65% with an interquartile range of [56,69] and extremes between 7% and 85%. LVEF was greater than 50% in 326 patients (73.9%). 83 patients (18.8%) had LVEF less than or equal to 35%.

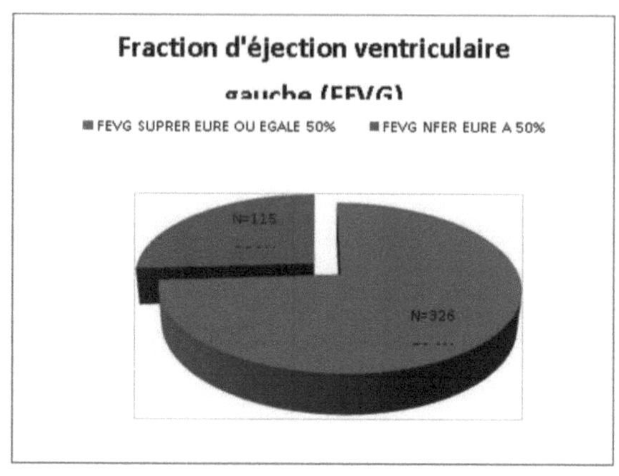

Figure 5: Distribution by left ventricular ejection fraction

1.8- Anti-aggregating and anticoagulant treatment :

- Long-term oral anticoagulant therapy with VKAs was prescribed in 73 patients (16.6%),
- Antiplatelet agents were observed in 90 patients (20.4% of

cases),

- 50 patients were on aspirin alone (11.3%), and 40 patients (9.1%) were on dual anti-platelet aggregation (aspirin and clopidogrel),

- Three patients, all with mechanical mitral prosthesis, received curative heparin therapy (0.7%) at a rate of 4 to 7mg/kg/day by electric syringe with an APTT of 60 to 92 seconds.

-

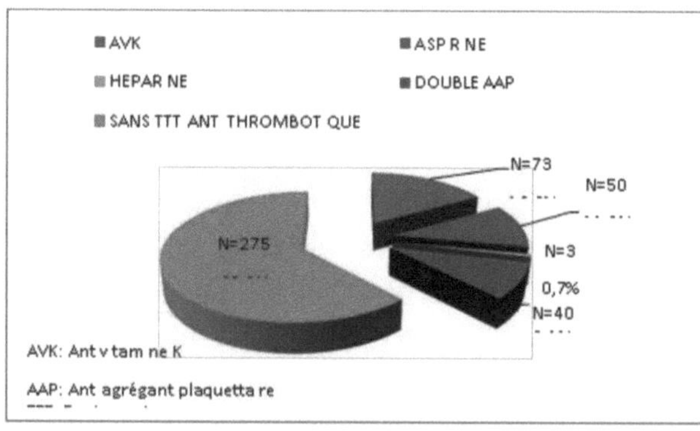

Figure 6: Distribution of anticoagulant and antiplatelet therapy

1.9- Characteristics related to the location

a- Type of device implanted :

359 patients (81.4%) were implanted with a pacemaker, and 82 patients (18.6%) were fitted with an ICD.

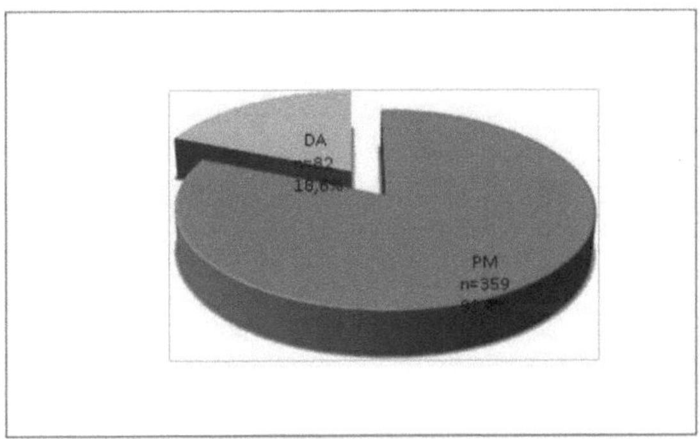

Figure 7: Distribution by type of device implanted

b- Indication

❖ **Pacemakers:** 359 patients were implanted with a pacemaker. The indications are distributed according to the following indications (table II)

Table II: Distribution by indication and type of pacemaker

Indication	Mono-Room	Double room	Triplechamber	TotalN (%)
2nd degree BAV and bradyarrhythmias	28 (25,7%)	32 (12,9%)	0 (0%)	60 (16,7%)
3rd degree AVB	68 (62,4%)	147 (59,3%)	0 (0%)	215 (59,9%)
Sinus Dysfunction	13 (11,9%)	69 (27,8%)	0 (0%)	82 (22,8%)
Resynchronization cardiac	0 (0%)	0 (0%)	2 (100%)	2 (0,6%)
Total by indication	109 (30,4%)	248 (69,1%)	2 (0,6%)	359

❖ **Implantable automatic defibrillators:** 82 patients were fitted with an ICD. The indications are detailed in Table III.

Table III: Distribution by indication and type of ICD

Indication	Mono-Room	Double room	Triple room	Total N (%}
Primary prevention	13 (54,2%)	28 (59,6%)	9 (81,8%)	50 (61,0%)
Secondary prevention	11 (45,8%)	19 (40,4%)	2 (18,2%)	32 (39,0%)
Total by indication	24 (5,4%)	47 (10,7%)	11 (2,5%)	82

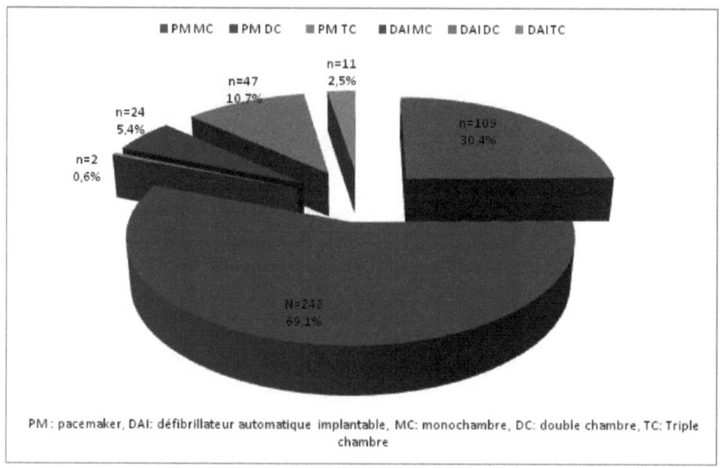

Figure 8: Distribution according to the type of implanted device c- First-time implantation versus re-implantation :

In our population, 25 patients had a box change (5.7%), divided into:

- seven patients with a single chamber pacemaker,
- 15 patients with a double chamber pacemaker,
- A single patient with a single chamber ICD,
- A single patient with a dual chamber ICD,
- A single patient with a triple chamber ICD.

Of these 25 patients, only two had more than two lead changes, both from a defibrillator. Four patients had an additional lead placement, three right ventricular and one atrial, all for lead wear (one for lead breakage, three for lead insulation erosion).

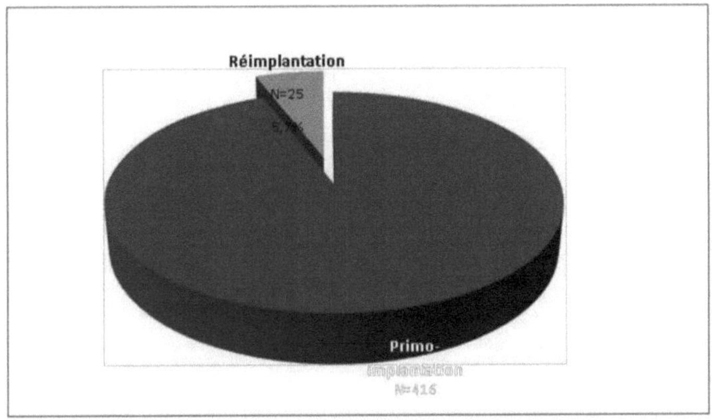

Figure 9: Distribution according to first implantation

d- Temporary electrosystolic drive :

In our population, 6 patients (1.4%) had a provisional electrosystolic pacing lead inserted while waiting for a definitive cardiac stimulation, without any complication. For five pacer-dependent patients who required a change of pacemaker, a provisional electrosystolic pacing lead was inserted via the right femoral route in these patients (1.1%) without any complication related to this procedure immediately or later.

e- Venous approach :

420 patients had at least one venous approach, 416 for primary implantation and 4 for reimplantation. The most frequent approach was the right subclavian route. Ten patients had an approach via the cephalic vein and the ipsilateral subclavian vein, 8 on the right side and 2 on the left side.

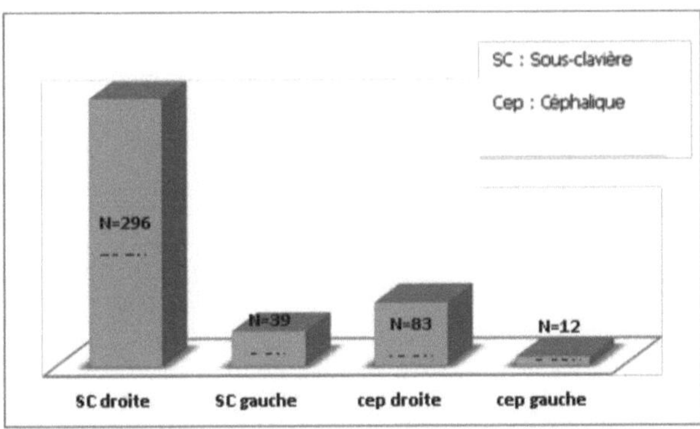

Figure 10 : Distribution according to the vascular approach f- Probes

728 probes were implanted, of which 209 were passive and 519 active, divided into:

❖ 420 VD probes of which 196 are passive (26.9%)

❖ 295 right atrial probes, all active (40.5%)

❖ 13 passive left ventricular leads (1.8%), 11 positioned at the level of the lateral vein, one at the level of a posterolateral coronary vein, and one at the level of an anterolateral vein.

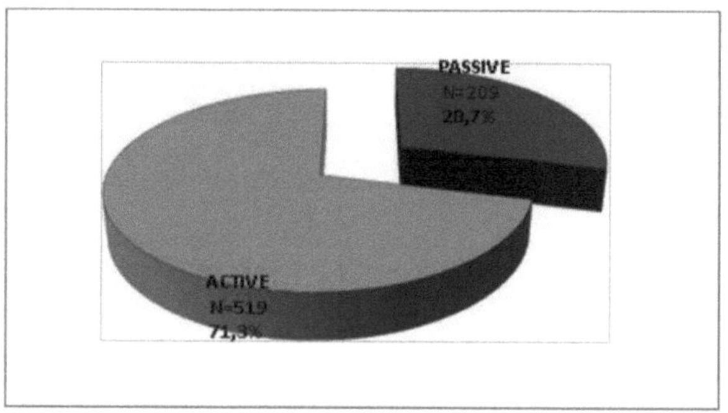

Figure 11: Distribution by probe attachment

g- Duration of the procedure

The median procedure time was 55 min, with an interquartile range of [45,65] and extremes between 35 and 310 min. Table IV summarizes the characteristics of the procedure time according to the implanted device.

Table IV: Duration of the procedure according to the device implanted

Implanted device	Duration of the procedure in minutes Median, interquartile range (or extremes when not defined}
PM single room	45 [35,50]
PM double room	65 [55,75]
PM triple room	127 [90,165] *
Single chamber DAI	55 [45,55]
DAI double room	65 [55,75]
DAI triple room	165 [155,175]

PM: pacemaker, ICD: automatic implantable defibrillator, *: extremes, interquartile range not defined

h- Length of hospitalization :

The median length of stay was 2 days with an interquartile range of [2,3] and extremes of 1 day and 10 days.

2 - EARLY COMPLICATIONS (<30 DAYS) :

a- Overall prevalence :

We counted 35 complications in 34 patients, i.e. an overall prevalence of 7.9%. 33 patients had a single complication and only one patient had two simultaneous complications.

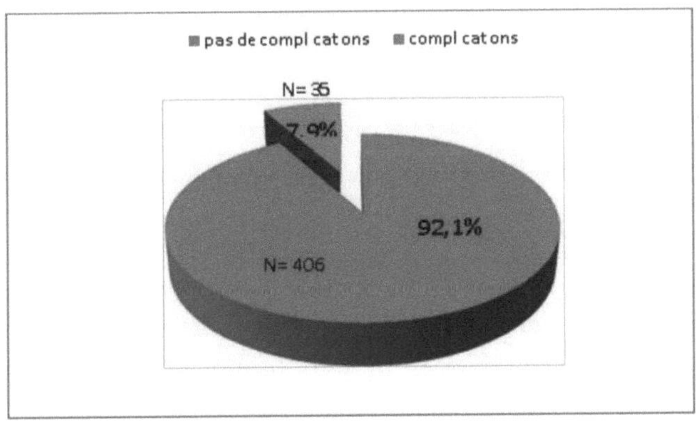

Figure 12: Overall prevalence of complications

b- Prevalence by type of complication :

b.1- Pneumothorax :

Pneumothorax was the most frequent complication. We counted 18 cases of pneumothorax, which corresponded to an overall prevalence of 4.1% and represented 51.4% of all complications. Taking into account the simple changes of the boxes, this rate became 4.3%. Only one patient presented a hemo-pneumothorax.

All patients who presented with a pneumothorax were approached by subclavian venous approach. 15 patients (88.2%) were drained in relation to a total pneumothorax, one of whom presented a suffocating obstructive pneumothorax complicated by cardio-circulatory arrest recovered after exsufflation. Two patients (11.7%) presented a partial pneumothorax which regressed after 7 days of rest without drainage.

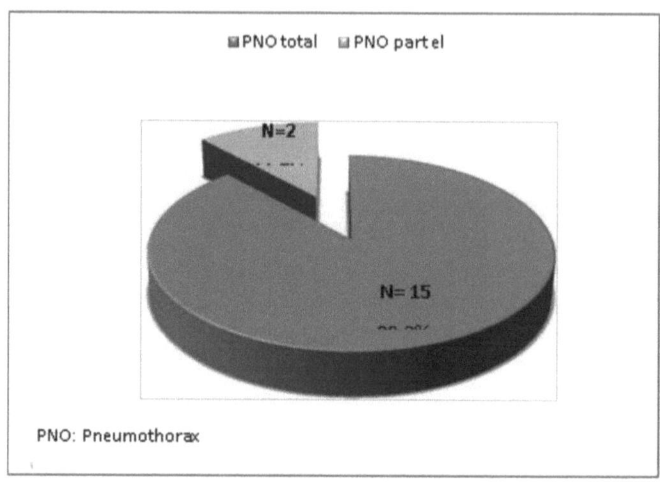

FIGURE 13: Distribution according to the type of pneumothorax b.2- Infection :

There were five cases of infection, all of them of the lodge, which represented a prevalence of 1.1% and 14.3% of all complications. No cases of endocarditis on catheter were retained. All these cases involved male patients. The bacteriological investigation was negative in four cases, and one case was associated with an infection by **Serratia Marescens** identified on the pus culture. Blood cultures were all negative and there were no suspicious images of vegetations on the probes in any of the patients. All these patients were put on anti-staphylococcal antibiotics for 7 days and then had an explantation of the box with extraction of the material on the 8th day, and reimplantation of the stimulator on the contralateral side on the same day, without complications. The patient who had been fitted with the defibrillator refused to undergo a new implantation.

b.3- Hematoma :

We found three cases of hematoma, all in patients with mechanical mitral prosthesis, which evolved well spontaneously. The prevalence was 0.7% which represented 8.6% of all complications. All patients were under curative unfractionated heparin.

b.4-Venous thromboembolic disease :

We reported one case of right jugular vein thrombosis and one case of non-fatal pulmonary embolism. The jugular thrombosis was not associated with ipsilateral subclavian vein thrombosis. It appeared to be secondary to difficulty in advancing the catheter through the right Pirogoff confluence. The overall prevalence was 0.5% or 5.7% of all complications.

b.5-Probe displacement :

We identified 3 cases of lead displacement; one for an atrial lead, a second for a right ventricular lead and a third for a left ventricular lead. All the patients were recovered within 2 to 48 hours with optimal repositioning of the leads. The prevalence was 0.7% or 8.6% of all complications.

b.6-Cardiac perforation:

Two cases of perforation were found. The first was a non-fatal perforation of the right ventricle without tamponade in a patient who underwent subsequent emergency surgery with removal of the lead and placement of an epicardial lead. In the second case, a patient presented a tamponade in relation to a perforation by the guidewire, complicated by death at D3 postoperatively.the prevalence was 0.5% which represented 5.7% of all complications.

b.7-Death :

In our study we recorded three deaths, which represented a rate of 0.7%. The causes of death were related to:

► a case of tamponade in a patient who had undergone a triple chamber pacemaker implantation and who was drained in emergency and then referred to cardiovascular surgery, whose intra-operative exploration did not reveal any perforation by the probes and who died at D3 post-op following a septic shock
► a case of electro-mechanical dissociation 18 hours after implantation of a single-chamber ICD in primary prevention of ischemic dilated cardiomyopathy without arguments in favor of cardiac perforation or pulmonary embolism (echography done two hours before death without arguments of right ventricular thrombosis, and post-mortem without visualization of a pericardial effusion),
► a case of acute lung edema complicating a tight aortic stenosis

calcified, occurring one hour after implantation.

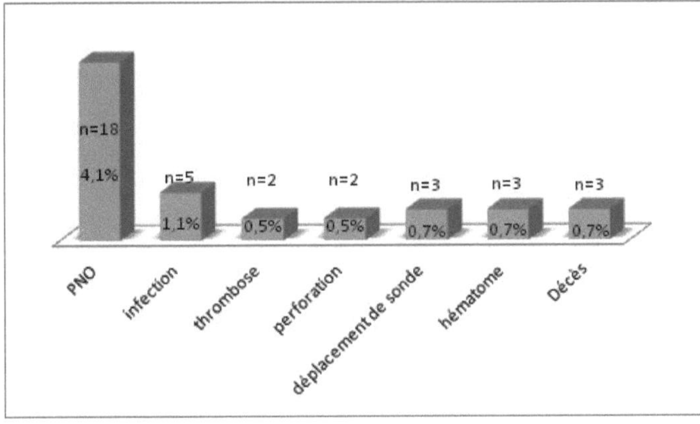

Figure 14: Distribution by type of complication

c- Time of occurrence of the complication:

23 patients had a complication on the day of implantation. The median time of occurrence of these complications was 1 day with an interquartile range of [1,27], and extremes between 1 and 28 days. The latest complication was a pacemaker box infection.

The occurrence of a complication increased the length of hospital stay by a median of 4 days with extremes between 2 and 8 days. (Length of hospital stay increased from 2 days with an interquartile range of (2-3)] without complication to 6 days with an interquartile range of (5-

11), p<0.001).

II- COMPARATIVE STUDY :

We subdivided our population into two groups:

- Group A: including patients without complications
- Group B: including the 34 patients with complication(s).

1- Univariate analysis:

1.1- Comparison according to epidemiological data :

a-   Age, gender, cardiovascular risk factors and history:

We found that complications were significantly associated with **diabetes (p=0.031}. Valve replacement and emboligic rhythm disorders** were close to the threshold of significance (p=0.07 and 0.10 respectively). Table V details these parameters.

Table V: Association between epidemiological factors and complications

	Group A N=407	Group B N=34	GOLD and its IC	p
Type Men Women	218 (53,6%) 189 (46,4%)	18 (52,9%) 16 (47,1%)	0,98 [0,51-1,87]	0.94 (NS)
HTA	265 (65,1%)	21 (61,8%)	0,98 [0,59-2,22]	0.71 (NS)
Diabetes	216 (53,1%)	22 (64,7%)	**2,15 [1,09-4,23]**	**0,031**
Dyslipidemia	123 (30,2%)	7 (20,6%)	1,61 [0,72-3,61]	0.24 (NS)
Dyspnea on exertion NYHA ≥2	159 (39,1%)	14 (41,2%)	0,92 [0,48-1,78]	0.81 (NS)
Active smoking	139 (34,2%)	10 (29,4%)	1,22 [0,60-2,49]	0.57 (NS)
COPD	14 (3,4%)	3 (8,9%)	0,41 [0,14-1,22]	0.13 (NS)
Valve replacement	17 (4,2%)	4 (11,8%)	3,05 [0,70-10,2]	0.07 (NS)

Embolism -related disorders	53 (13,0%)	9 (26,5%)	2,50 [0,79-6,79]	0.10 (NS)
IRC	11 (2,7%)	2 (5,9%)	0,49 [0,13-1,82]	0.26 (NS)
Valvulo pathy	31 (7,6%)	6 (17,6%)	2,51 [0,97-6,51]	0.51 (NS)
Dysthyr oidism	13 (3,2%)	1 (2,9%)	0,92 [0,02-6,49]	1.00 (NS)
Weight (kg}	64 [55,74]	65 [60,72]	-	0.70 (NS)
Age (years)	66,5±11,1	66,2±11,3	-	0.96 (NS)
FEVG	65 [45,69]	60 [35,70]	-	0.62 (NS)

COPD: chronic obstructive pulmonary disease, CKD: chronic renal failure, Kg: kilogram, OR: Odds ratio, CI: confidence interval of the Odds ratio at 95%, p: significance level. For Gaussian variables, we show their means and standard deviations, and for non-Gaussian variables we calculated the medians and the interquartile range (in square brackets).

b- Anticoagulant and antiaggregant treatment:

A significant association was found between complications and **curative heparin therapy (p<0.001}.** The association between complications and anticoagulants (anti-vitamin K and/or heparin) was very close to significance (p=0.051). The use of anti-vitamin K alone or anti-platelet agents was not statistically associated with complications.

Table VI: Association between antiaggregant and anticoagulant treatments with complications

	Group A N=407	Group B N=34	GOLD and its IC	p
HNF	0 (0%)	3 (8,8%)	5,14* [5,14-Inf]	<0,001
VKA without UFH	63 (15,5%)	7 (20,6%)	0,73 [0,33-1,60]	0.43 (NS)
Anticoagulants (VKA and/or UFH}	63 (15,5%)	10 (29,4%)	2,27 [0,92-5,22]	**0,051** (limit)
AAP	80 (19,7%)	10 (29,4%)	1,70 [0,70-3,87]	0.19 (NS)

UFH: unfractionated heparin, VKA: vitamin K antagonist, PAA: antiplatelet agent, OR: Odds Ratio, CI: 95% confidence interval, p: degree of significance, Inf: infinite bound, *: lower bound value. The values in square brackets are the bounds of the confidence interval.

1.2- Comparison according to the data of the implementation procedure

The **subclavian** vascular **approach** was significantly associated with complications **(p<0.001)**. We did not find a statistical association with device size (ICD vs. PM) or re-intervention for device change. The duration of the procedure was not statistically related to complications. There was no statistically significant association between the number of leads and the method of their fixation with complications.

Table VII: Association between procedural data and complications

	Group A N=407	Group B N=34	GOLD and its IC	p
SC vs CEP	337 (82,8%)	19 (55,9%)	**3,80**	<0,00
	70(17,2%)	15 (44,1%)	[1,84-	**1**
			7,84]	
Probe	162 (24,4%)	21 (39,7%)	0,64	0.12 (NS)
passive vs. active	503 (75,6%)	42 (67,7%)	[0,37- 1,12]	
PM vs DAI	74 (18,2%)	8 (12,5%)	0,74	0,44
	333 (81,8%)	26 (87,5%)	[0,31- 1,66]	(NS)
Change of Housing	25 (6,1%)	0 (0%)	-	0.24 (NS)
Numbers	2 [1,2]	2 [2,2]	-	0,25
Duration of the procedure (min)	55 [45,65]	62,5 [55,75]	-	0,16

SC: subclavian valve, POC: cephalic line, PM: pacemaker, ICD: implantable cardioverter defibrillator, mn: minutes, OR: crude Odds Ratio if calculable, (-): not calculable, CI: 95% confidence interval, p: significance level. The values in square brackets are relative to the bounds of the interquartile range. The bounds of the confidence interval are in bold brackets.

1.3-Factors associated with the occurrence of pneumothorax :

We found 4 parameters significantly related to the occurrence of pneumothorax:

✓ **Dyslipidemia** was statistically associated with a high prevalence of pneumothorax (100% vs 0%, **p=0.002**),

✓ The **rhythm disorders** were significantly related to pneumothorax (50% vs 5.5%, **p=0.007**),

✓ **VKAs** were statistically associated with a lower risk of pneumothorax (5.9% vs 56%, **p=0.002**),

✓ The **subclavian route** was associated with a significantly higher rate of pneumothorax (81% vs 33%; **p=0.005**).

2- Multivariate analysis

We adopted a logistic regression model without constant which allowed us to identify independent predictive factors for the occurrence of complications.

These factors are:

❖ **Curative heparin therapy (p<0.001),**
❖ **The subclavian route (p=0.009},**
❖ **Diabetes (p=0.038}.**

Table IX summarizes the adjusted odds ratios and the degree of significance.

TableVIII: Independent Predictive Factors and Adjusted ORs for Complications

	GOLD	Lower terminal of the IC	Top terminal of the IC	p
HNF	9,90	4,37	22,22	<0,001
Track SC	2,76	1,29	5,92	0,009
Diabete s	2,23	1,04	4,77	0,038

CI: confidence interval, p: significance level

For pneumothorax, the only independent factor for the occurrence of pneumothorax was the subclavian route with an adjusted OR of 25.64 ([0.78, 1000], p=0.068).

DISCUSSION

Permanent cardiac pacing is one of the most important medical innovations of the 20th century. Initially designed for the prevention of sudden death from syncopal complete atrioventricular block, its indications were expanded to include sinus dysfunction. With the advent of cardiac defibrillation, the morbidity and mortality associated with severe ventricular rhythm disorders and conduction disorders was greatly reduced.The expansion of indications for cardiac resynchronization has improved the vital and functional prognosis in certain patient populations. Atrioventricular block is the primary reason for implantation in the United States[1]. 1] Indeed, more than 50% of American patients have been implanted for atrial dysfunction. Technological advances have made it possible to extend the indication for cardiac pacing to obstructive hypertrophic heart disease and severe systolic heart failure.Despite preventive measures, this therapy is still burdened by a rate of complications that has remained stable for several years [4-12]. However, the follow-up of patients with pacemakers suffers from several shortcomings, firstly concerning the standardisation of telemetric monitoring and secondly concerning the management of complications. The prevention of complications requires a pre- and post-operative evaluation of the particular needs of each patient and an individual optimization of the pacing method.

I-Main results of our study :

Our study revealed the following results:

• The overall prevalence of early complications, occurring within one month of pacemaker and defibrillator implantation, was 7.9%,
• There is no statistically significant difference between complications after pacemaker or defibrillator implantation,

• There was no statistically significant increase in the rate of these complications between primary and reimplantation,
• The median time of occurrence of complications was 1 day. The occurrence of a complication statistically significantly increased the length of stay by a median of 4 days,

• The most frequent complication was pneumothora (4.1%), followed by infection of the lodge (1.1%),

• The independent predictors of complication were curative heparin therapy (OR=9.9 (4.37 - 22.22), p<0.001), subclavian line (OR=2.76(1.29 -5.92), p=0.009), and diabetes (OR=2.23 (1.04 -4.77), p=0.038)
• The only independent predictive factor for pneumothorax was the subclavian route with OR=25.64 but with a very wide confidence interval ((0.78-1000), p=0.068).

II-Epidemiological profile :

1- Age:

The existence of a linear relationship between age and the occurrence of onductive disorders is well established [14-23]. Indeed, the age group most concerned by this pathology is between 50 and 80 years [14,21,22]. In our work, the average age of the patients studied was 66.5 11.1 years. The age range ≥ 75 years represented 36.3% of our population.

In a Spanish registry reported by Samartinetal [24] which included 11,648 patients, the mean age was 76.8 years. Bouraoui et al [12] collected 234 patients whose mean age was 69.5 years.Slimane and Ben Ameur published in 2002 the results of the only Tunisian multicentric study on 35 double chamber pacemakers and the average age of their population was 58.4 ± 16 years. The increase in life expectancy has led to an increase in the number of elderly patients fitted with pacemakers. Indeed, more than half of the permanent pacemaker recipients are elderly patients aged under 7 years[15,16,19,21-26]. Link et al [25] pooled data from theCTOPP [35], UKPACE [36] and a Danish study [14].A total of4814 patients were included in this analysis, with a mean follow-up of 5.1 a The mean age was 76 years and 43% were femaleAn early complication occurred in 5.1% of patients ≥75 years compared with 3.4% of patients aged < (=0.006). Early complications were higher in patients receiving pacemakers with atrial leads in both age groups (<75 years: 4.6% versus 2.4%; ≥75 years: 6.6% versus 3.7%). However, the relative risk is not influenced by age.Nowak et al [26] in a German multicenter retrospective study conducted from 2003 to 2006 studied different indications according to ageThey found that AF and conductive disturbances increase with age, whereas sinus dysfunction was less frequent in older subjects.   There was no statistically significant difference in the rate of complications according to age.The distribution of the different indications for definitive cardiac pacing are comparable to those found in the literature [26]. The mean age of patients with high-grade AVB was 70.6±13 years, whereas patients with sinus dysfunction had a mean age of 67, ± 13 years (p=0.027).The mean age of patients implanted with a single-chamber PM was significantly higher than that of patients implanted with a dual-chamber PM (75.0 years vs 64.6 years; p=0.024).Schmidteal [28] studied the clinical characteristics and survival in implanted patients aged ≥ 80 years.In this German study conducted between 1971 2000, 1588 patients aged ≥ 80 years were included.PM implantation in this age group accounted for 3of a total number of implantations.The prognostic factors identified were:Exemasculin (RR–1.20; CI=1.04 to 1.40; p≤0.2], PM VVI [RR=1.42; CI=1.12 to 1.81; p≤ 0.005) and age ≥ 85years at implantation, were identified as being associated with poorer long term survival.   However, none of these parameters predicted outcome or choice of PM type.

2- Gender:
In the international literature [27,37-40], there is a clear male predominance. In the Tunisian study of 2002 [11], there were 176 men and 177 women, and in our work the sex ratio was close to 1.
Nowak et al [39] in a German multicenter retrospective study, 7826 primary implanted patients were collected between 2003 and 2006 In this study, men had more BA and less sinus dysfunction than women.Women had more short-term complications than men regardless of age and type of implanted MP (5.8% vs. 4.7%; OR=1.3; CI=1 to 1.5). The most frequent complications were pneumothorax (0.74% in women vs. 0.35% in men; OR=2; p<0.01; 95% CI 1.39 to 3.24) and hematoma loge (0.87 in females vs 0.58 in males; OR=1.49; 95% CI 1.05 to 2.11; p<0.01).   Concerning long-term follow-up, women had a significantly better survival than men despite an older age at implantation.Several authors [27,29,30,34,37-39,41] have identified male gender as a risk factor for long-term mortality. In our work, the rate of diabetes, hypertension, dyslipidemia and obesity was higher in women, without reaching statistical significance.   On the other hand, the female sex was not associated with an increased risk of early complications.

3-   Cardiovascular risk factors :

Given the advanced age of the population interested in cardiac pacing, it is common to find the existence of several cardiovascular risk factors. This situation partly explains the occurrence of clinical events during follow-up. 53.4% of the patients surveyed by Bouraoui et al [12] were found to have hypertension. In our work, hypertension was present in 64.9% of the patients, and diabetes in 19.7% of the population studied by Bouraoui et al [12]. 29.5% of the population was diabetic in Hajlaou's study [9].The diabetic population represented 54% of the patients in our series.Bouraoui et al [12] noted dyslipaemia in only

3.4% of the patients, whereas we counted 29.5% of dyslipaemics.Obesity was found in 9.4% of the cases in the work of Bouraoui and 28.9% of our patients.

III-Clinical data :

In our series, lipothymia and syncope were noted respectively in 50.6% and 24.5% of cases.In the Tunisian series, the main reason for consultation was lipothymia encountered in 44 to 64% of patients, followed by syncope in 26 to 35% of patients [8,9,11,12].Our findings are consistent with the Tunisian series.

IV-   Indications for definitive cardiac pacing and defibrillation :

The indications for definitive cardiac pacing imply a comprehensive and logical diagnostic approach, with not only a precise diagnosis of the conductive disorder, but also the demonstration of a causal link between this anomaly and the symptoms described by the patient. Finally, proof or strong presumption of chronicity and irreversibility of the conductive disorder must be considered [3-7]. These indications are well codified and regularly updated by the learned societies [3-6]. In clinical practice   ,   the   main pathologies for pacemaker implantation are AVB and sinus dysfunction. In our work, high-grade AVB represented 57.0% of the indications. Sinus dysfunction was the reason for definitive pacing in 26% of cases.   Table IX shows the indications in different studies in the literature.

Table IX: Indications for pacing in the literature

Indications Series	High-grade AVB	Sinus Dysfunction
Mourali (1997)[8]	58,1%	19,4%
Lamas et al (1998)[45]	49,0%	43,0%
Connolly et al (2000)[46]	51,0%	33,0%
Hajlaoui (2001) [9]	66,0%	18,0%
Slimane et al (2002)[11]	80,0%	16,0%
Proclemeretal (2009)[39]	51,7%	28,8%
Samartin et al (2011)[14]	55,6%	20,2%
Bouraoui (2011) [12]	74,4%	17,1%
Sdiri et al (2013) [13]	74,5%	16,0%
Our series	**57,0%**	**26,0%**

NB: the figures in brackets refer to the year of publication of the series

In Tunisia, the main indications for definitive cardiac pacing remain high-grade AVB followed by sinus dysfunction [8,9,11,12].In Western series, sinus dysfunction becomes the first reason for implantation.This difference can be explained by the fact that sinus dysfunction, often paroxysmal, can go unnoticed on the surface ECG. For economic reasons, these examinations are less practiced in our country, which could explain this low rate of diagnosed sinus dysfunction. For the indications of cardiac defibrillation, the two indications of primary and secondary prevention are classically opposed.The large MUST MADITII and SCDHef trials have shown the considerable contribution of this device in the reduction of sudden death [7].In our country, the most frequent indication is that of secondary prevention, biased by essentially economic constraints.

V- Complications:

The increase in the number of pacemaker implants and in the number of indications has been accompanied by an increase in the risk of intra- and postoperative complications [2,7]. The morbidity and mortality depend mainly on the clinical status of the patient, the conditions of implantation and the occurrence of infection of the pacing device [2,14,18].A strategy should therefore be proposed based on prevention and anticipation of complications on the one hand, and on regular monitoring of definitive pacemakers on the other [2,47,48].The literature is well provided for the evaluation of the prevalence of early complications of pacemakers or the IDA [5,19-32], but it seems difficult to provide information on the association of two devices simultaneously and the evaluation of complications limited to the first month, as well as the predictive factors associated with them.

A- Early complications :

In our study we found that the prevalence of complications in the first 30 days after implantation of a cardiac pacemaker was 7.9 of the total number of patients implanted with pneumothor as the predominant complication which accounted for 51.4% of the total complications.One of the first studies of the prevalence of complications related to cardiac pacing is that of Pearson and colleagues in 1989[49]. The rate of complications during the period 1982-1986 was between 0.2 and 10.2%, of which approximately 1/3 was related to pneumorax.TheFOLLOWPACE study[41] is a multicenter prospective registry conducted in23 Dutch centers,from January200 November 2007This cohort included1517 patients who had just had their first definitive cardiac stimulus implantatio for symptomatic bradycardia. Short-term complications [$\leq$ 2 months]were reported in 188 patients or 12.4% of the study population.The study by Kirkfeldt et al in 2013 as part of the national registry in Denmark found an overall complication rate over the first six months of 9.5% [19].In the study by Sdiri et al, the early complication rate, assessed at one month after implantation, was 6.9, mainly haemorrhagic and/or thrombo-embolic complications in 2.1% of cases [13].Ludwig et al found a complication rate of 12%. They grouped pneumothorax in the category of mechanical complications which also included wave dysfunction.Cantillon et al found an overall complication rate of 8.9%, dominated by lead displacement (3.7%), pneumothorax (3%), hemothorax (1.4%) and infection (1.2%) [52].In a recent study, Defay investigated the complication in patients exclusively equipped with an implantable automatic defibrillator. It found an overall complication rate of 9.8%, which was significantly higher for dual-chamber ICDs compared to single-chamber ICDs (1vs 9%). These complications were dominated by lead displacement (4.2%) and pneumothorax was 0.6% [53].

a- Pneumothorax:

We found in our work that pneumothorax was the most frequent complication, in association with the subclavian approach. In Tunisian series, this rate varies between 0 and 1.6% [8,11,14,50]. Pakarinen found a rate of 1.9 [21] while Udo found a rate of 2.2% [41].Kirkfeldt reported that 1.6% of these patients developed a pneumothorax [1 while Cantillon who has the largest series of patients (7207) found 2.9% pneumothorax with a rate that rises to 6.6% in case of associated hemothorax [52].

b- Lodge hematoma:

In our series, 3 patients with a mitral prosthesis who were under curative heparin therapy developed hematoma of the lodge, which corresponds to a rate of 0.7%. In Tunisian series, this rate ranged from 2 to 9.7% [8,11,14,50].In international series, this rate is higher than our result. Pakarinen found a rate of 3.2% [21].   Udo found a rate of 4.7% [41].Kirkfeldt reported that 2.5% of his patients developed a hematoma of the lodge, almost half of which required a reoperation [19].Cantillon found only 0.1% of hematomas of the lodge with a rate that rises to 6.6% in the case of associated hemothorax [52].

c- Moving the probes :

In our work, the rate of displacement of the atrial lead was 0.2% (one patient).   For ventricular leads, we noted a displacement rate of 0.5% (two patients). The overall rate of lead displacement was 0.7%.In the Tunisian series, the rate oscillated between 1.3 and 9.7% [8,11,14,50].In the FOLLOWPACE study (Udo et al), the rate of complications related to pacing leads was 5.5%. The most frequent complication was lead displacement with a rate of 3.3%[41].The passive fixation ventricular lead had the highest rate of displacement (3.9%) while the active ventricular lead was displaced in only 1.9% of cases (p=0.059).In the work of Kirkfeldt et al [1], lead-related complications were most common (3.6%) and occurred equally in ventricular atrial leads (2.3 vs 2.2%; p=NS).Pakarinen et al found an early lead displacement rate of 3.7% with no statistically significant difference between atrial and ventricular leads (2.7% vs. 2.2%; p=0.65) [21].Kirkfeldt reported that 2.7% of patients had lead displacement [19] while Cantillo found 3.5% lead displacement [52]. The table below summarizes the early complications detailed in the various Tunisian and international studies.

Table X: Early complications in the literature

Series	N	Overall rate	Pneumothorax	Hematoma of the lodge	Displacement of the probe
Mourali (1997} [8]	37	-	0%	9,7%	9,7%
Slimane [11]	353	14,6%	0,3%	3%	9%
Sdiri(2013} [14]	188	6,9%	1,6%	2,1%	1,6%
Chouchen (2007} [50]	234	10%	0%	5%	1,3%
Pakarinen (2010}[21]	825	13,5%	1,9%	3,2%	3,7%
Udoetal (2012} [41]	1517	12,4%	2,2%	4,7%	3,3%
Kirkfeldt et al(2013} [19]	5918	9,5%	1,6%	2,5%	2,7%
Cantilloet al(2014} [52]	72071	8,9%	2,9% (+3,7%)	0,1%	3,5%
Our series	441	7,9%	4,1%	0,7%	0,5%

N: number of patients included in the series, figures in brackets are for the year of publication, overall rate: rate of all complications in the study population. The figures in italic brackets are those related to pneumothorax. (-): no information.

d- Early infectious complications:

Although there is a need for more information on pacemaker implant techniques and antibiotic prophylaxis [51-56], infections of pacemaker devices are not essential [57,59].The learned societies regularly publish recommendations to help the practitioner diagnose these infectious complications, standardize their management, and improve preventive measures [61,62].Pacing device infective endocarditis is a well-established but fortunately rare complication [59-64]. The clinical picture may be evident in the presence of a skin fistula with purulent secretion, long-term fever associated with a biological inflammatory syndrome. Transesophageal echocardiography may show images of vegetations at the level of the probes. The evolution may be complicated by septic pulmonary embolism. The clinical picture is often insidious with fever and altered general condition. Blood cultures are rarely positive and echocardiography is not very helpful. The germ responsible is often a very slowly multiplying saprophytic staphylococcus epidermidis, which has been shown to vary according to the authors from 0.1% to 20[56]. Infections occurring within 2 months after implantation are considered to be serious and constitute 25% of infections on pacing equipment.The distinction between these two entities is not unanimously accepted by the scientific community. Table XI summarizes the incidence of early infectious complications in the different series.

Table XI: Early infectious complications in the literature

Series	Early infectious complications
Mourali (1997} [8]	3,2%
Slimane (2002} [11]	2,3%
Catanchin (2007} [66]	1,6%
Chouchen (2008} [50]	3,6%
Pakarinen (2010}[21]	1,9%
Sdiri (2013} [13]	1,6%
Kirkfeldtetal (2013} [19]	0,8%
Cantillonetal(2014} [52]	1,2%
Our series	1,1%

Figures in brackets are for the year of publication

Johansen et al[5 are interested in infectious complications after implantation of definitive cardiac pacing devices. In this prospective study, 46299 implantation procedures (of which 44630 were post-implantation and166 were device replacements) were included during a period of19200. During the follow-up, 596 PM extractions for suspected infection (345 post-implantation and 251 post- replacement) were identified. Infection was confirmed by bacteriological criteria in 461 patients (77.3%). Street factors for infection were: re-interventions, male, young age, and lack of antibiotic prophylaxis.Pakarinen et al[21] reported the results of a retrospective study that focused on early complications (<3 months). This study was conducted in Finland during the year 2000 and included 825 procedures. Infectious complications were identified in 1.9% of the patients, including perficial wound infections that responded rapidly to antibiotic treatment, 7 endocarditis from foreign material (1.2%) that required explantation and 4 compartment infections. Catanchina [6] reported the results of a prospective study that included 14 patients. The authors found 3 cases of infection, 24 of which were bacteriologically confirmed endocarditis [an incidence of 1.6%]. The rate of infection in patients who had a primary implantation was 0.88% vs. 3.99% in patients who underwent reoperation (OR= 4.7; 95% CI=2.1 to 10.6; p=0.001). In this study, advanced age, diabetes, duration of the procedure, and operator inexperience were the predictive factors of infection.In the majority of cases, the treatment of endocarditis in pacing equipment requires the removal of the pacing equipment (limbs and leads) associated with prolonged antibiotic therapy. The evolution is often favourable with no recurrence in 10% of cases in the study by Catanchin [66].Athan et al [63] prospectively collected 2760 cases of infective endocarditis on pacing material.The in-hospital mortality rate was 14.7%.In our series, we found cases (0.50% of the population) of infective endocarditis occurring late after a pacing procedure. This high figure can be explained by a relatively low rate of extraction of implanted material (one patient out of two, i.e. 50% of cases), and the late diagnosis.

e- Early thromboembolic complications:

Thromboembolic disease is one of the most serious complications after pacemaker implantation[65-6 has been shown to be associated with an increased risk of thromboembolic events (TE) during follow-up.In our series, the rate of thromboembolic complications was 0.5%. In our series, the thromboembolic complication rate was 0.5%. There were two patients, one with jugular thrombosis resulting in failed ond implantation requiring reoperation, and one with pulmonary embolism, both of which progressed well on anticoagulant therapy. Cantillon found a rate of these complications of 0.5% [52].Che et al[69] analyzed the risk factors for TE events in 4 consecutive patients with pacemaker implantation.TE events were identified in 11 patients (2.%) within 7 days of pacemaker implantation.Four patients (36.%) died as a result of TE implantation. The analysis revealed that an age of 4 years (OR=4,; P=0.031), hypertension (OR=3.59P=0.028), diabetes (OR=8.89;

P<0,001),	lamaladiecoronaire	(OR=4.8	P=0.005),	fibrillation
auriculaire	[FA](OR=5.68;	P=0.006)the	FAchronic	persistent

(OR=10.; p<0.001)e history of stroke

The prevalence of TE events in the perioperative period was not significantly different between patients with single and dual chamber pacemakers.To this end, a Polish study by Elakowski et al[7] enrolled 81 patients with pacemakers who had a 3.0% rate of symptomatic thrombosis in the study population:a history of myocardial infarction temporary cardiac pacing, ultra ventricular arrhythmias venous anomaly, NYHA class III and IVu history infection and smoking. In patients who had more risk factors, a near 100% probability of occurrence of venous obstruction was observed.In the Tunisian series[8,9,11,13,50] crude data on thromboembolic complications are not available.

f- Reintervention:

Inourseries, 3 patients (8.8%) had a re-intervention, all for catheter displacement.Concerning early re-interventions, Ud et al [41] reported that the main cause was catheter displacement.Of the patients who had early complications, one third required re-intervention.According to Eberhardt et al [18], the rate of complications requiring reoperation was 4.5%, of which 7% were early complications (<3 months). In the Followpa study [41], the independent predictive factors were the occurrence of cardiac and congestive heart failure, the use of antagonists, the subclavian venous access, and active fixation atrial leads. In addition, the amount of central line activity did not appear to affect the rate of short-term complications (RR=1 p=0.78).

g- Perforation :

We have two cardiac perforations that correspond to a complication rate of 0.5%.The Tunisian series did not include this complication.In the FOLLWPACE registry, only 0.13 complications were associated with cardiac perforation [41].akarinen found a rate of 0.7% of cardiac perforation of which 1 ¾ were complicated by tamponade [21].irkfeldt reported that 0.8% of these patients had a cardiac perforation [19].Cantillon found in a series of 389 patients which corresponded to a rate of 0.56% [52].

h- Deaths :

The death rate in the Tunisian periphery is higher than in the international series, and the mortality rate was 0.7%. The only study that detailed this result was Kirkfeld, who found a one-month all-cause mortality rate of 1.4% [19].

B- Predictive factors of complications :

We foundcomm independent predictive factors for the occurrence of complications, and curativehaprino-therapydiabetesandvoisclaviclepremiefactlyassociatedwithhaematolysisandinfectionandthird with pneumothorax. No conclusive association was found between the complications and :
-    Age,

-    Gender,

-    Chronic renal failure,

-    The number of probes,

-    Implantation of an ICD,

-    Re-installation or change of box,

-    The duration of the procedure,

We were unable to find a statistical association between the epidemiological factors studied and the occurrence of infectious complications. Camus et al report that diabetes, corticosteroids and anticoagulants are associated with infection in the space between the implant and the patient, without specifying the early occurrence of this complication [65].Catanchint found that the association between the occurrence of infection and the duration of the operation[66] and the use of provisional electrosystolic training seems to increase this risk significantly [64,66,67]. In our series, given the low rate of infectious complications (1.1%), we lacked the power to carry out a statistical analysis to identify the factors that predict complication. For venous thrombosis, Korkeila and Chen noted that this complication was frequently associated with low weight, supraventricular arrhythmias and a history of pulmonary disease [69,70]. In multivariate analysis, Kristensen found that persistent atrial fibrillation was independently associated with subclavian thrombosis (OR=9; P<0.001)[71].The history of myocardial infarction, supraventricular arrhythmia, anomalous vein infection, and suffocating cardiac disease were predictive factors for the occurrence of this complication [72].With regard to anticoagulation, the current data in the literature underline the frequent association of haematolloge with curative heparin therapy [73-83]. This risk seems to be lower with antiplatelet agents and vitamin K antagonists [81-83].For direct oral anticoagulants, the data in the literature are currently scarce. For the size of the device, the studies seem to favour a high complication rate for implantable automatic defibrillators compared with pacemakers [84,88]. In our series, we did not find any significant difference in these two situations.

- Prolonged antibiotic prophylaxis over 48 hours,

- The preparation of the intra or sub pectoral lodge,

- The size of the defibrillators is getting smaller and smaller

- For perforation, we found a prevalence of 0.2%.   The data in the literature give a rate of between 0 and 6.4% but count both early and late perforations [86,89].   There does not seem to be a factor associated with this complication, even if it is anatomical, relating to the thickness of the free wall of the right ventricle [86].

VI- Limitations of the study and perspectives :

Our study was retrospective and monocentric, which could induce a selection bias.The number of some complications was low, which hindered a robust statistical analysis and induced a lack of power. We did not analyze the relationship of these complications with the provisional electro-systolic training leads because of the low number of placements of these leads.The confidence interval of the Odds Ratio of complications was very scattered secondary to the relatively low number of complications inducing a systematic uncertainty of the estimation of the latter.he number of certain complications such as hematoma of the lodge or death was very low inducing a lack of power in the statistical analysis. We found as a factor associated with the complications, diabetes, probably by its interaction with the infectious risk We propose a therapeutic trial comparing two different regimens of antibiotic prophylaxis in diabetic patients fitted with an implantable cardiac device.he reduction of the hematoma rate under heparin therapy would be achieved through the use of an electric scalpel.This hypothesis could also be the subject of a therapeutic trial protocol.ith regard to the most frequent complication which is pneumothorax, we recommend a systematic recourse to the cephalic route. he creation of a national register including all the implantations practiced in Tunisia, whether in public or private structures, will allow to access the exact rate of complications and to identify after a more robust statistical analysis the predictive factors of complications which will allow to refine the management of this category of patients, and to establish national recommendations relating to the management of our implanted patients.

REFERENCES

1.   Trohman RG, Kim MH, Pinski SL. Cardiac pacing the state of the art. Lancet. 2004;364(9446):1701-19.

2.   Wilkoff BL, Auricchio A, Brugada J, Cowie M, Ellenbogen KA , Gillis AM et al. HRSEHRA Expert Consensus on the Monitoring of Cardiovascular Implantable Electronic Devices (CIEDs) Description of Techniques, Indications, Personnel, Frequency and Ethical Considerations. Heart Rhythm. 2008;5(6):907-25.

3.   Epstein AE, Dimarco JP, Ellenbogen KA, Estes NA [3rd], Freedman RA, Gettes LS et al. ACC/AHA/HRS 2008 Guidelines for Device-Based Therapy of Cardiac Rhythm Abnormalities. J Am Coll Cardiol. 2008;5:934-55.

4.   Brignole M, Auricchio A, Baron-Esquivias G, Bordachar P, Boriani G, Breithardt OA, et al. 2013 ESC guidelines on cardiac pacing and cardiac resynchronization therapy: the task force on cardiac pacing and resynchronization therapy of the European Society of Cardiology (ESC). Developed in collaboration with the European Heart Rhythm Association (EHRA). Europace. 2013;15:1070-1118.

5.   Dickstein K, Vardas PE, Auricchio A, Daubert JC, Linde C, McMurray J et al. 2010 Focused Update of ESC Guidelines on device therapy in heart failure An update of the 2008 ESC Guidelines for the diagnosis and treatment of acute and chronic heart failure and the 2007 ESC guidelines for cardiac and resynchronization therapy. Eur Heart J. 2010;31:267787.

6.   Kusumoto FM, Schoenfeld MH, Barrett C, Edgerton JR, Ellenbogen KA, Gold MR et al. 2018 ACC/AHA/HRS Guideline on the Evaluation and Management of Patients With Bradycardia and Cardiac Conduction Delay: A Report of the American College of Cardiology/American Heart Association Task Force on Clinical Practice Guidelines and the Heart Rhythm Society. J Am Coll Cardiol. 2019;74(7):e51-e156.
7.   Hayes DL, Furman S. Cardiac pacing how it started, where we are, where we are going.J Cardiovasc Electrophysiol. 2004;15(5):619-27.
8.   Mourali MS. Definitive cardiac pacing by double chamber pacemaker. Experience of the cardiology department EPS Charles Nicolle. Thesis of Doctorate in Medicine Tunis, 1997. 143p.

9.   Hajlaoui N. Definitive dual chamber cardiac pacing: Indications and follow-up,

Experience of the cardiology department of the military hospital of Tunis [Thesis]. Medicine: Tunis; 2000. 132p.

10. Ben Ameur Y, Ouchallal K, Hmam M, Terras K, Battikh K, Slimane ML. Indications for definitive cardiac stimulation. Tunis Med. 2001;79:561-68.

11. Slimane ML, Ben Ameur Y. The dual chamber cardiac pacing. A multicenter study A propos of 353 pacemakers. Tunis Med. 2002;80(10):624-7.
12. Bouraoui H, Trimech B, Chouchene S, Mahdhaoui A, Ernez Hajri S, Jeridi G, et al. Permanent cardiac pacing about 234 patients. Tunis Med. 2011;89(7):604-9.

13. Sdiri W, Marouf A, Mbarek D, Ben Slima H, Mokaddem A, Ben Ameur Y, et al. Results of cardiac pacing: About 188 patients. Tunis Med. 2013;91(6):396-401.

14. Aggarwal RK, Connelly DT, Ray SG, Ball J, Charles RGl. Early complications of permanent pacemaker implantation no difference between dual and single chamber systems.

Br Heart J. 1995;73(6):571-5.
15. Andersen HR, Nielsen JC, Thomsen PE, Thuesen L, Mortensen PT, Pedersen AK. Long-term follow-up of patients from a randomised trial of atrial versus ventricular pacing for sick-sinus syndrome. Lancet.1997;350(9086):1210-6.

16. Deniz HB, Caro JJ, Ward A, Moller J, Malik F. Economic and health consequences of managing bradycardia with dual-chamber compared to single-chamber ventricular pacemakers in Italy. J Cardiovasc Med. 2008;9(1):43-50.
17. D'Souza R, Dawson F, Kerr F. Experience of a small British pacing centre between 1994and 2000 some answers to the problem of low UK implantation rates. Scott Med J. 2001;46(6):173-5.

18. Eberhardt F, Bode F, Bonnemeier H, Boguschewski F, Peters W et al. Long term complications in single and dual chamber pacing are influenced by surgical experience and patient morbidity. Heart. 2005;91(4):500-6.

19. Kirkfeldt RE, Johansen JB, Nohr EA, Moller M, Arnsbo P, Nielsen JC. Risk factors for lead complications in cardiac pacing A population-based cohort study of 28,860 Danish patients. Heart Rhythm. 2011;8(10):1622-8.
20. Kiviniemi MS, Pirnes MA, Eranen HJ, Hartikainen JE. Complications related to permanent pacemaker therapy. Pacing Clin Electrophysiol. 1999;22(5):711-20.

21. Pakarinen S, Oikarinen L, Toivonen L. Short-term implantation-related complications of cardiac rhythm management device therapy a retrospective single-centre 1-year survey. Europace. 2010;12(1):103-8.
22. Van Eck JWM, Van Hemel NM, Zuithof P, Van Asseldonk JPM, Voskuil TLHM, Grobbee DE et al. Incidence and predictors of in-hospital events after first implantation of pacemakers. Europace. 2007;9(10):884-9.

23. Bayata S, Yeşil M, Arikan E, Postaci N, Berligen R, Ceylan O et al. Retrospective analysis of 1650 permanent pacemaker implantations experience over two different consecutive time periods in a single cardiology clinic. Anadolu Kardiyol Derg. 2010;10(2):130-4.

24. Coma Samartfn R, Sancho-Tello de Carranza MJ, Ruiz Mateas F, Del Ojo Gonzalez JL, Fidalgo Andres ML. Spanish Pacemaker Registry. Seventh official report of the Spanish Society of Cardiology Working Group on Cardiac Pacing (2009). Rev Esp Cardiol. 2010;63(12):1452-67.

25. Link MS, Estes NA 3rd, Griffin JJ, Wang PJ, Maloney JD, Kirchhoffer JB et al. Complications of dual chamber pacemaker implantation in the elderly. Pacemaker Selection in the Elderly (PASE) Investigators. J Interv Card Electrophysiol. 1998;2(2):175-9.

26. Nowak B, Misselwitz B. Effects of increasing age onto procedural parameters in pacemaker implantation results of an obligatory external quality control program. Europace. 2009;11(1):75-9.
27. Pyatt JR, Somauroo JD, Jackson M, Grayson AD, Osula S, Aggarwal RK et al. Long-term survival after permanent pacemaker implantation analysis of predictors for increased mortality. Europace. 2002;4(2):113-9.

28. Schmidt B, Brunner M, Olschewski M; Hummel C, Faber TS, Grom A et al. Pacemaker therapy in very elderly patients long-term survival and prognostic parameters. Am Heart J. 2003;146(5):908-13.

29. Armaganijan LV, Toff WD, Nielsen JC, Andersen HR, Connolly SJ,Ellenbogen KA, et al. Are elderly patients at increased risk of complications following pacemaker implantation A meta- analysis of randomized trials. Pacing Clin Electrophysiol. 2012;35(2):131-4.

30. Jahangir A, Shen WK, Neubauer SA, Ballard DJ, Hammill SC, Hodge DO et al. Relation between mode of pacing and longterm survival in the very elderly. J Am Coll Cardiol. 1999;33(5):1208-16.

31. Stambler BS, Ellenbogen KA, Orav EJ, Sgarbossa EB, Mark Estes NA, Rizo-Patron C et al. Predictors and clinical impact of atrial fibrillation after pacemaker implantation in elderly patients treated with dual chamber versus ventricular pacing. Pacing Clin Electrophysiol. 2003;26(10):2000-7.

32. Steinbach M, Douchet MP, Bakouboula B, Bronner F, Chauvin M. Outcome of patients aged over 75 years who received a pacemaker to treat sinus node dysfunction. Arch Cardiovascular Dis. 2011;104(2):89-96.

33. Stevenson RT, Lugg D, Gray R, Hollis D, Stoner M, Williams JL. Pacemaker implantation in the extreme elderly. J Interv Card Electrophysiol. 2012;33(1):51-8.

34. Udo EO, van Hemel NM, Zuithoff NPA; Kelder JC, Crommentuijn HA, Koopman-Verhagen AM et al. Long-term outcome of cardiac pacing in octogenarians and nonagenarians. Europace. 2011;14(4):502-8.

35. Kerr CR, Connolly SJ, Abdollah H, Roberts RS, Gent M, Yusuf Set al. Canadian Trial of Physiological Pacing Effects of physiological pacing during long-term follow-up. Circulation. 2004;109(3):357-62.

36. Toff WD, Camm AJ, Skehan JD. Single-chamber versus dual-chamber pacing for highgrade atrioventricular block. N Engl J Med. 2005;353:145-55.

37.   Brunner M, Olschewski M, Geibel A, Bode C, Zehender M. Long-term survival after pacemaker implantation. Prognostic importance of gender and baseline patient characteristics. Eur Heart J. 2004;25:88-95.

38. Irnich W. Gender differences in pacemaker therapy. Europace. 2010;12:1202-3.

39. Nowak B, Misselwitz B, Erdogan A, Funck R, Israel CW, Olbrich HG et al. Do gender differences exist in pacemaker implantation--results of an obligatory external quality control program. Europace. 2010;12:210-5.

40. Roeters Van Lennep JE, Zwinderman AH, Roeters Van Lennep HW, Van Hemel NM, Schalij MJ, Van der Wall EE. No gender differences in pacemaker selection in patients undergoing their first implantation. Pacing Clin Electrophysiol. 2000;23:1232-8.

41. Udo EO, Zuithoff NPA, van Hemel NM, De Cock CC, Hendriks T, Doevendans PA, et al. Incidence and predictors of short- and long-term complications in pacemaker therapy The FOLLOWPACE study. Heart Rhythm. 2012;9:728-35.

42. Kirkwood G, Fox DJ, Brown BD. Bradycardia pacing. Medicine. 2014;42:615-9.

43. Merin O, Ilan M, Oren A, Fink D, Deeb M, Bitran D et al. Permanent pacemaker implantation following cardiac surgery indications and long-term follow-up. Pacing Clin Electrophysiol. 2009;32:7-12.

44. Proclemer A, Ghidina M, Gregori D, Facchin D, rebellato L, Zakja E et al. Trend of the

main clinical characteristics and pacing modality in patients treated by pacemaker data from the Italian Pacemaker Registry for the quinquennium 2003-07. Europace. 2010;12:202-9.

45. Beck H, Boden WE, Patibandla S, Kireyev D, Gutpa V, Campagna F, et al. 50th Anniversary of the first successful permanent pacemaker implantation in the United States historical review and future directions. Am J Cardiol. 2010;106:810-8.

46. Lamas GA, Lee K, Sweeney M, Leon A, Yee R, Ellenbogen K et al. The mode selection trial (MOST) in sinus node dysfunction design, rationale, and baseline characteristics of the first 1000 patients. Am Heart J. 2000;140:541-51.

47. Connolly SJ, Kerr CR, Gent M, Roberts RS, Yusuf S, Gillis AM et al. Effects of physiologic pacing versus ventricular pacing on the risk of stroke and death due to cardiovascular causes. Canadian Trial of Physiologic Pacing Investigators. N Engl J Med. 2000; 342:1385-91.

48. Van Eck JWM, Van Hemel NM, de Voogt WG, Meeder JG, Spierenburg HA, Crommentuyn H et al. Routine follow-up after pacemaker implantation frequency, pacemaker programming and professionals in charge. Europace. 2008;10:832-7.

49. Parsonnet V , Bernstein AD, Lindsay B. Pacemaker-implantation complication rates: an analysis of some contributing factors. J Am Coll Cardiol. 1989;13(4):917-21.

50. Chouchène S. Definitive cardiac pacing indications and results. Experience of the cardiology department of the Farhat Hached hospital in Sousse [Thesis]. Medicine. Sousse, 2007. 140p.

51. Ludwig S, Theis C, Wolff C, Nicolle E, Witthohn A, Gatte A. Complications and associated healthcare costs of transvenous cardiac pacemakers in Germany.   J Comp Eff Res. 2019;8(8):589-97.

52. Cantillon DJ, V Exner DV, Badie N, Davis K, Yan Gu N, Nabutovsky Y, et al. Complications and Health Care Costs Associated With Transvenous Cardiac Pacemakers in a Nationwide Assessment. JACC Clin Electrophysiol. 2017;3(11):1296-1305.

53. Defaye P, Boveda S, Klug D, Beganton F, Piot O, Narayanan K, **et al**. Dual- vs. single-chamber defibrillators for primary prevention of sudden cardiac death: long-term follow-up of the Implantable Automatic Defibrillator-Primary Prevention registry. Europace. 2017;19(9):1478-84.

54. Wranicz JK, Chudzik M, Cygankiewicz I, Klimczak A, Kaczmarek K, Maciejewski M et al. Pacing and sensing disturbances in patients with DDD pacemakers in the early period after implantation. Acta Cardiol. 2006;61(3):289-94.

55. Bertaglia E, Zerbo F, Zardo S, Barzan D, Zoppo F, Pascotto P. Antibiotic prophylaxis with a single dose of cefazolin during pacemaker implantation incidence of long-term infective complications. Pacing Clin Electrophysiol. 2006;29:29-33.

56. Cengiz M, Okutucu S, Ascioglu S, Sahin A, Aksoy H, Deveci OS et al. Permanent pacemaker and implantable cardioverter defibrillator infections seven years of diagnostic and therapeutic experience of a single center. Clin Cardiol. 2010;33:406-11.

57. Filali T, Fehri W, Ben Moussa M, Chriaa S, Barakett N, Gommidh M et al. Infective endocarditis on probe of pacemaker. Tunis Med. 2009;87:610-15.

58. Johansen JB, J0rgensen OD, M0ller M, Arnsbo P, Mortensen PT, Nielsen JC. Infection

after pacemaker implantation infection rates and risk factors associated with infection in a population-based cohort study of 46299 consecutive patients. Eur Heart J. 2011;32:991-8.

59. Mokaddem A, Bachraoui K, Sdiri W, Kachboura S, Boujnah MR. Pacemaker infections. Tunis Med. 2002;80:509-14.

60. Mounsey JP, Griffith MJ, Tynan M, Gould FK, MacDermott AF, Gold RG, Bexton RS. Antibiotic prophylaxis in permanent pacemaker implantation a prospective randomised trial. Br Heart J. 1994;72:339-43.

61. Habib G, Lancelotti P, Antunes MJ, Bongiorni MG, Casalta JP, Del Zotti F et al. 2015 ESC Guidelines for the management of infective endocarditis: The Task Force for the management of Infective Endocarditis of the European Society of Cardiology (ESC). Eur Heart J. 2015;36(44):3075-128.

62. Baddour LM, Epstein AE, Erickson CC, Knight BP, Levison ME, Lochhart PB, et al. Update on Cardiovascular Implantable Electronic Device Infections and Their Management A Scientific Statement From the American Heart Association. Circulation. 2010;121:458-77.

63. Athan E, Chu VH, Tattevin P, Selton-Suty C, Jones P, Naber C et al. Clinical haracteristics and outcome of infective endocarditis involving implantable cardiac devices. JAMA. 2012; 307(16):1727-35.

64. Camus C. Serious infections related to pacemakers and implantable defibrillators. Reanimation. 2008;17:225-32.
65. Camus C, Donal E, Bodi S, Tattevin P. Implantable pacemaker and defibrillator-related infections. Med et Mal Infect. 2010;40:429-39 .
66. Catanchin A, Murdock CJ, Athan E. Pacemaker Infections A 10-Year Experience. Heart Lung Circ. 2007;16:434-9.

67. Knigina L, Kühn C, Kutschka I, Oswald H, Klein G, Haverich A et al. Treatment of patients with recurrent or persistent infection of cardiac implantable electronic devices. Europace. 2010;12:1275-81.

68. Lepillier A, Otmani A, Waintraub X, Ollitrault J, Le Heuzey JY, lavergne T. Temporary transvenous VDD pacing as a bridge to permanent pacemaker implantation in patients with sepsis and haemodynamically significant atrioventricular block. Europace. 2012;14:981-5.

69. Chen S, Liu J, Pan W, Liu S, Su Y, Bai J, et al. Thromboembolic events during the perioperative period in patients undergoing permanent pacemaker implantation. Clin Cardiol. 2012;35:83-7.

70. Korkeila P, Nyman K, Ylitalo A, Koistinen J, karjalainen P, Lund J et al. Venous obstruction after pacemaker implantation. Paceing Clin Electrophysiol. 2007;30:199-206.

71. Kristensen L, Nielsen JC, Mortensen PT; Pedersen OL, Pedersen AK, Andersen HR. Incidence of atrial fibrillation and thromboembolism in a randomised trial of atrial versus dual chamber pacing in 177 patients with sick sinus syndrome. Heart. 2004;90:661-6.

72. Lelakowski J, Domagała TB, Cieśla-Dul M, Rydlewska A, Majewski J, Piekarz J, et al. Association between selected risk factors and the incidence of venous obstruction after pacemaker implantation demographic and clinical factors. Kardiol Pol. 2011;69:1033-40.

73. Amara W, Ben Youssef I, Monsel F, Sergent J. Antiplatelet agents increase hemorrhagic risk in patients undergoing a cardiac pacemaker or ICD implantation. Ann Cardiol Angeiol. 2011;60:267-71.

74. Kutinsky IB, Jarandilla R, Jewett M, Haines DE. Risk of hematoma complications after device implant in the clopidogrel era. Circ Arrhythm Electrophysiol. 2010;3:312-8.

75. Przybylski A, Derejko P, Kwaśniewski W, Urbanczyk-Swic D, Zakrzewska J, Orszulak W, et al. Bleeding complications after pacemaker or cardioverter-defibrillator implantation in patients receiving dual antiplatelet therapy Results of a prospective, two-centre registry. Neth Heart J. 2010;18:230-5.

76. Samama CM, Bastien O, Forestier F, Denninger MH, Isetta C, Juliard JM et al. Antiplatelet agents in the perioperative period expert recommendations of the French Society of Anesthesiology and Intensive Care (SFAR) 2001-summary statement. Can J Anaesth. 2002;49(6):S26-35.

77. Tompkins C, Cheng A, Dalal D, Brinker JA, Leng CT, Marine JE et al. Dual antiplatelet therapy and heparin "bridging" significantly increase the risk of bleeding complications after pacemaker or implantable cardioverter-defibrillator device implantation. J Am Coll Cardiol. 2010;55:2376-82.

78. Thal S, Moukabary T, Boyella R, Shanmugasundaram M, Pierce MK, Thai H et al. The relationship between warfarin, aspirin, and clopidogrel continuation in the peri-procedural period and the incidence of hematoma formation after device implantation. Pacing Clin Electrophysiol. 2010;33:385-8.

79. Hammerstingl C, Omran H. Perioperative bridging of chronic oral anticoagulation inpatients undergoing pacemaker implantation--a study in 200 patients. Europace. 2011;13:1304-10.

80. Amara W, Ben Youssef I, Kamel J, Ghrissi I, Faron M, Khouadja A et al. Evaluation of the bleeding risk of different perioperative anticoagulation protocols during primary implantation or replacement of a pacemaker or defibrillator analysis of a cohort of patients in a general hospital. Ann Cardiol Angeiol. 2009;58:265-71.

81. Amara W, Ben Youssef I, Bonny A, Faron M, Monsel F, Sergent J. Implantation of pacemakers and defibrillators under antivitamin K does not increase bleeding risk. Ann Cardiol Angeiol. 2010;59:255-9.

82. Cheng A, Nazarian S, Brinker JA, Tompkins C, Spraag DD, Leng CT et al. Continuation of warfarin during pacemaker or implantable cardioverter-defibrillator implantation: a randomized clinical trial. Heart Rhythm. 2011;8:536-40.

83. Ahmed I, Gertner E, Nelson WB, House CM, Dahiya R, Anderson CP et al. Continuing warfarin therapy is superior to interrupting warfarin with or without bridging anticoagulation therapy in patients undergoing pacemaker and defibrillator implantation. Heart Rhythm. 2010;7:745-9.

84. Poole JE, Gleva MJ, Mela T, Chung MK, Uslan DZ, Borge R et al. Complication rates associated with pacemaker or implantable cardioverter-defibrillator generator replacements and upgrade procedures results from the REPLACE registry. Circulation. 2010; 122:1553-61.

85. Tibi T, Moceri P, Martin Teule C, Berkane N, Talbodec A, Tannous J, et al. Local registry of pacemaker implantations proposals to decrease infectious risk. Ann Cardiol Angeiol. 2006;55:339-41.

86. Schwerg M, Stockburger M, Schulze C, Bondke H, Poller WC, Lembcke A et al. Clinical, anatomical and technical risk factors for postoperative pacemaker or defibrillator

lead perforation with particular focus on myocardial thicknesses. Pacing Clin Electrophysiol. 2014;37:1291-6

87. Olsen T, orgensen OD, Nielsen JC, Thogersen AM, Philbert BT, Johansen JB. Incidence of device-related infection in 97 750 patients: clinical data from the complete Danish device- cohort (1982-2018). Eur heart J. 2019;40:1862-69.

88. Nowak B, Tasche K, Barnewold L, Heller G, Schmidt B, Bordignon S, et al. Association between hospital procedure volume and early complications after pacemaker implantation: results from a large, unselected, contemporary cohort of the German nationwide obligatory external assurance programme. Europace. 2015;17:787-93.

89. Vamos M, Erath JW, Benz AP, Bari Z, Duray GZ, Hohnloser SH. Incidence of Cardiac Perforation With Conventional and With Leadless Pacemaker Systems: A Systematic Review and Meta-Analysis. J Cardiovasc Electrophysiol. 2017;28(3):336-346.

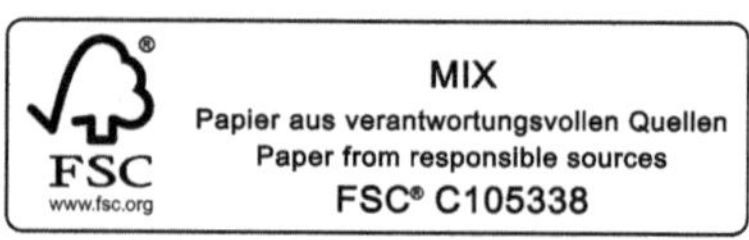

Printed by Books on Demand GmbH, Norderstedt / Germany